The Rough Guide to the Foundation Programme

2nd Edition, July 2007

Produced by:

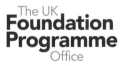

The UK
**Foundation
Programme**
Office

Edited by: Carrie G Moore

Acknowledgements:
The Rough Guide was produced with the help of many people and we would like to thank
them for their contributions, particularly Dr Ajay Bedi, Charlene Binding, Janet Brown,
Dr Stuart Carney, Dr Elizabe   Blackpool, Fylde and Wyre NHS   University Hospitals Leicester NHS
Trust for some excellent phi   Library   David Graham, Shannon Guy,
Professor Shelley Heard, Dr.   ng, Dr Ed Neville, Dr Scott Oliver,
Professor Elisabeth Paice, Su   am Sullivan plus many more.

Published by TSO (The Stationery Office) and available from:

Online
www.tsoshop.co.uk

Mail, Telephone, Fax & E-mail
TSO
PO Box 29, Norwich, NR3 1GN
Telephone orders/General enquiries: 0870 600 5522
Fax orders: 0870 600 5533
E-mail: customer.services@tso.co.uk
Textphone 0870 240 3701

TSO Shops
16 Arthur Street, Belfast BT1 4GD
028 9023 8451 Fax 028 9023 5401
71 Lothian Road, Edinburgh EH3 9AZ
0870 606 5566 Fax 0870 606 5588

TSO@Blackwell and other Accredited Agents

Published for the Department of Health under licence from the
Controller of Her Majesty's Stationery Office.

First published 2007

ISBN 978 0 11 703780 9

610.695 071 M00

Table of contents

Foreword   iv

Introduction   v

Chapter 1: Applying to the Foundation Programme   1

Chapter 2: Before you start   5

Chapter 3: Foundation year one (F1)   7

    The induction   8

    The placements   8

    Your study time   10

    Assessment   11

    Your Foundation Learning Portfolio   17

    Becoming a fully registered doctor   34

Chapter 4: Foundation year two (F2)   35

    The placements   36

    Study leave   40

    Assessment   41

    Your Foundation Learning Portfolio   41

Chapter 5: Life after foundation training   43

Chapter 6: Careers advice   47

Chapter 7: What else?   51

    Flexibility   53

    Location   57

    Trainees in difficulty   59

    Who's who?   63

    Further information   71

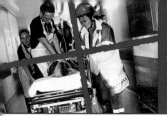
Dear colleague

As a doctor in the UK, you can look forward to receiving some of the best work-based medical education and training in the world. This guide tells you what to expect in your first two years working and learning in the health service.

The Foundation Programme was introduced in August 2005 to provide a stepping stone for junior doctors from medical school to specialty/GP training. The training you receive through the Foundation Programme will be structured, supervised and assessed against standards set out in the *Foundation Programme Curriculum*. The aim is to ensure you are equipped with the skills, attitudes and aptitudes that all doctors must possess for a career in the NHS.

It will embrace all key professional skills you need to ensure a patient gets the best possible care, including communications skills and multi-disciplinary team-working, in addition to clinical skills. Over the two years you will maintain a portfolio of achievements that demonstrates your progress in each of these areas.

The General Medical Council (GMC) has overall responsibility for your education during the first year of foundation training. The Postgraduate Medical Education and Training Board (PMETB) then becomes responsible for setting the standards of training from your second foundation year through specialty/GP run-through training and beyond.

The Foundation Programme as a whole is administered by the UK Foundation Programme Office, which is responsible to all four UK health departments. A website has been developed for medical students, foundation doctors and other interested parties, which contains all the information available on the Foundation Programme, including the curriculum and this Rough Guide (www.foundationprogramme.nhs.uk).

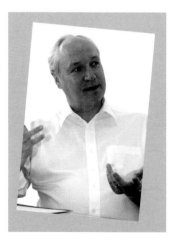

I wish you every success as you embark on your professional practice, and extend a warm welcome to the Foundation Programme.

Professor Derek Gallen
National Director,
UK Foundation Programme Office

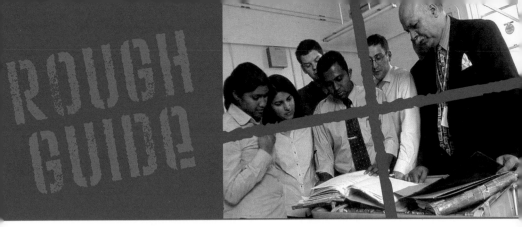

Introduction

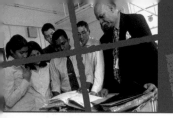

What is the Foundation Programme?

Your F1 post in the Foundation Programme will be the first medical job you have after you graduate. All medical school graduates must undertake, and complete, the Foundation Programme in order to work as a doctor in the UK.

It is typically made up of six, four-month placements over two years, and forms a bridge between medical school and specialty training. Your placements provide a safe environment to put in practice what you have learned at medical school, while giving you the additional skills, knowledge and experience needed to begin specialty or GP training.

The Rough Guide

This guide explains how the Foundation Programme works, and will help you get the most out of your first two years of clinical practice. It covers a range of topics including your application to the Foundation Programme; how you progress through F1 and F2; advice on completing your assessments; and advancing to specialty training. It also covers career advice and what to do if things are not going well in your placement.

The guide has been written for both final year medical students and foundation doctors, with contributions from foundation doctors, clinical tutors, educational supervisors, postgraduate deans and others involved in foundation programmes across the UK. It isn't exhaustive, but provides a good starting point to find out more about how your first two years of training will work. If you want to know the details of absolutely everything about the Foundation Programme, refer to the Operational Framework for Foundation Training.

If you want to share your experiences and/or give us advice about how to make it better, visit **www.foundationprogramme.nhs.uk** to find out how to contribute to future editions of the *Rough Guide*.

How does foundation training work?

As you would expect, the Foundation Programme is designed so you can gain basic competence in core clinical skills as well as other professional skills like communication, teamwork and the use of evidence and data. You will be expected to demonstrate increasingly sophisticated skills in these areas throughout the Foundation Programme, well beyond what you learned in medical school.

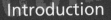
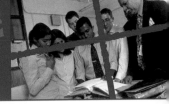

Your first foundation placement will usually commence in early August after medical school graduation. You will rotate to your next placement every 3, 4, or 6 months (depending on how your foundation school sets up your programme), and over the two years you will build up a portfolio of assessments and achievements as you gain more experience and acquire new competences. Part of this will involve asking your colleagues to assess your clinical and professional skills in a range of settings while you work.

At the end of each year, you must demonstrate that you have met the standards of competence set out in the *Foundation Programme Curriculum* (June 2007). There are a range of assessment tools you can use to prove your competence and they are detailed later in this guide.

Once you have successfully completed your first foundation year (F1), you will receive full registration by the GMC. Once you have successfully completed your second foundation year (F2), you will receive a Foundation Achievement of Competence Document (FACD). In order to work as a doctor in the UK, you must complete the Foundation Programme.

Throughout the whole programme, and as you progress through specialty/GP training and beyond, you will continue to gain new competences which you should add to your portfolio. Your portfolio shows evidence of the competences you have achieved in different areas and it will stay with you for the duration of your career.

What else can I expect?

You will be responsible for your own learning, making sure your assessments are completed, attending the structured learning sessions, organising any "tasters" (usually a week spent in a specialty you would not otherwise experience as a foundation doctor) and keeping your portfolio up to date.

Learning on the job is a key feature of the Foundation Programme, and you have lots of ground to cover in these first two years. Besides formal teaching sessions, you should consider every activity a chance to learn something new. Clerking patients, presenting on ward rounds and attending outpatients all add to your collection of knowledge. Always be on the lookout to add to your portfolio of competences and developing new clinical skills. For some competences, you may learn as much from nurses and non-clinical members of your healthcare team as from the senior doctors. Each day will bring many opportunities to learn. Grasp every chance you are given.

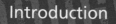

In each placement, you will have a named senior doctor as your educational supervisor. Their job is to help you through your training programme and to support your day-to-day learning. The precise arrangements will vary by foundation school. In some case, your educational supervisor could remain the same for the entire programme, in others the educational supervisor may change with each placement. But you will always be supported to ensure that you have good clinical supervision and a structured educational experience.

Who will organise my foundation training programme?

All of your postgraduate training is organised by your postgraduate deanery and will be managed through foundation schools. For more information on foundation schools, turn to page 64.

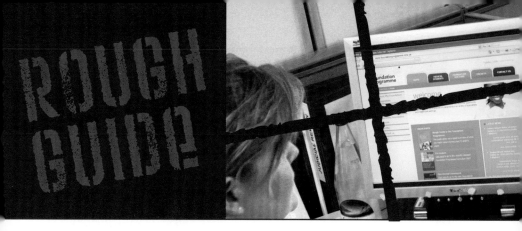

Chapter 1
Applying to the Foundation Programme

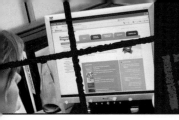

The application process

You will make a single online application to the Foundation Programme. As part of your application, you will rank the foundation schools you are interested in order of preference. You will be able to see the types of programmes they offer before you rank them.

You are responsible for completing and submitting your own application. Your medical school does not do this on your behalf. However, they will contact you with specific details on how and when to apply. Alternatively, go to www.foundationprogramme.nhs.uk for further details.

Although placements will vary, you will have exposure to the clinical and educational environments necessary for you to get all the competences required for you to complete foundation training.

One of the main aims of foundation training is to give you the opportunity to experience as wide a range of specialties and clinical settings as possible, in order to help inform your future career choice and provide you with a broad range of skills.

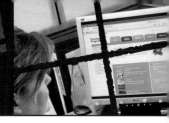

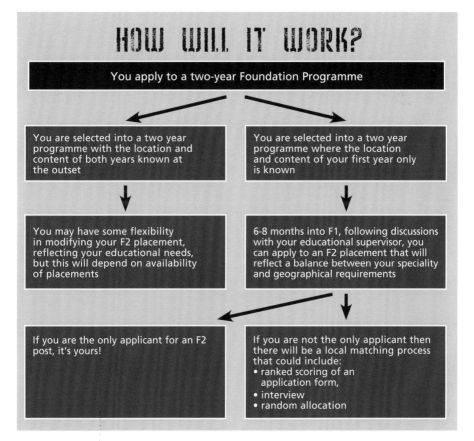

HOW WILL IT WORK?

You apply to a two-year Foundation Programme

You are selected into a two year programme with the location and content of both years known at the outset

You are selected into a two year programme where the location and content of your first year only is known

You may have some flexibility in modifying your F2 placement, reflecting your educational needs, but this will depend on availability of placements

6-8 months into F1, following discussions with your educational supervisor, you can apply to an F2 placement that will reflect a balance between your speciality and geographical requirements

If you are the only applicant for an F2 post, it's yours!

If you are not the only applicant then there will be a local matching process that could include:
• ranked scoring of an application form,
• interview
• random allocation

The application

You will fill out a standardized application form, along with all other final year UK, EEA and international medical school students. All EEA and UK medical students are treated equally in the application process and are competing for a limited number of places, so fill out your application carefully as you will not automatically get a place on the Foundation Programme.

There is a national person specification which sets out the knowledge, skills and attributes you need in order to become a foundation doctor. Each application

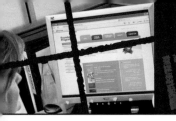
will be scored by a panel (including at least one senior doctor) against standardised scoring criteria. Your overall score will consist of an academic score provided by your medical school and the score relating to your application answers. The score provided by your medical school will give you points based upon the academic quartile you fit into. For example, you will receive a certain number of points for being in the top 25% of your class, another for falling between 25% - 50%, and so on.

You will need to identify two referees to support your application. They should be hospital consultants or practising GPs who can give their views on your previous performance. References will be used as part of the pre-employment checks once you have been offered a job and will not be included in the application scoring process.

What happens if I don't want the programme I am offered?

Successful applicants will be allocated to one foundation school only, and then to one programme only. Wherever possible, this will be done taking into account your declared preferences on your application form. If you decline your allocated foundation school (or programme allocation within that foundation school), this will mean you are withdrawing from the process altogether, and will not be able to begin the Foundation Programme that year.

The offer of a programme is not the same as the offer of a job.

If your application is successful, you are allocated a Foundation Programme place through the foundation schools. Once you have confirmed acceptance of your programme, the local healthcare organisation commence with pre-employment checks. Once they are satisfied, they will offer you a contract of employment.

Pre-employment checks

Pre-employment checks are carried out by employers. These checks may include Criminal Records Bureau (CRB) checks (England) or, in Scotland, Disclosure Scotland and Occupational Health Checks. In Northern Ireland, pre-employment checks are carried out by NIMDTA.

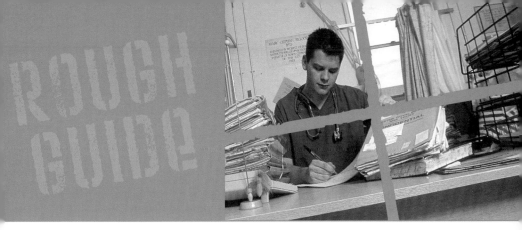

Chapter 2
Before you start

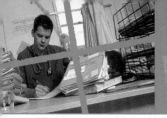
Provisional registration with the GMC

Before you can start work as an F1 doctor, you must be provisionally registered with the GMC. During your final year, the GMC visits your medical school and provides you with information about how to apply for provisional registration. Once you've passed your exams and paid a fee, your registration will automatically be activated.

Applying for provisional registration

a. **Go to www.gmc.org.uk and login to MyGMC.** Once you receive your graduation certificate, login to MyGMC (the secure area of the GMC website), to complete the application for provisional registration. The PIN code and password required to enter this section will be sent to you by the GMC after they visit your campus. Take this opportunity to ensure that all your details on MyGMC are correct – this is your last chance to change them easily. If you have forgotten your login details, you can contact the GMC. However, keep in mind that it may take up to five working days to receive them.

b. **Complete a fitness to practise declaration.** You must complete a fitness to practise declaration. The Registrar has the discretion to request additional information or evidence to ensure the integrity of the medical register. Requests for additional information may include a request to submit a recent (less than six months old) Criminal Records Bureau (CRB) report. The CRB report may take at least six to eight weeks to arrive.

c. **Pay for your registration.** MyGMC enables you to pay the £100 provisional registration fee online. It can be paid up to three months before you begin your F1 post.

It is crucial that you do not undertake medical work without registration! If you do, you will not be legally covered and any mistake could lead to a financial cost to you (not a good idea!).

Your university supplies the GMC with a list of successful graduates, so you will not need to send the GMC your certificate to finalise your registration.

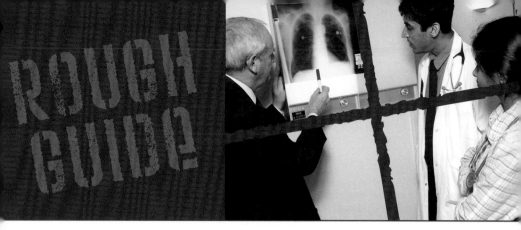

Chapter 3
Foundation year one (F1)

The induction

Before you start your first placement, there will be an induction course at your workplace. As well as receiving information about the hospital, your timetable and what is expected of you, you will be advised of the contact details of your educational supervisor and of the careers advice that is available locally.

Some rotations offer six months of medicine and six months of surgery but most foundation schools have already moved to offering three, 4-month attachments.

Both surgical and medical attachments are required for GMC registration.

Your F1 year will:

1. make sure you can put the knowledge, skills and attitudes you learnt as a student into practice as a doctor (as outlined in *The New Doctor*)

2. equip you with new knowledge and skills whilst supporting your professional development.

The placements

Your F1 placements will be determined by the post or programme for which you are selected. In addition to medicine and surgery, your post may include any of the 65 recognised specialties such as:

- haematology
- infectious diseases
- dermatology
- gynaecology
- anaesthetics
- ENT
- paediatrics
- acute stroke medicine

This list is far from complete but does give you an idea of the possible specialties that may be available to you. All jobs will enable you to work towards the Foundation Programme competences.

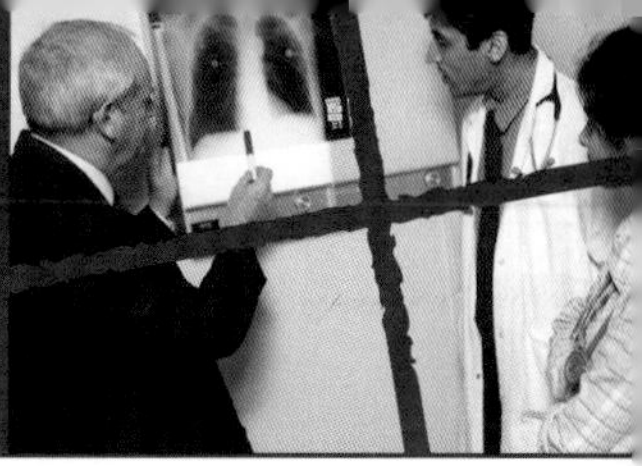

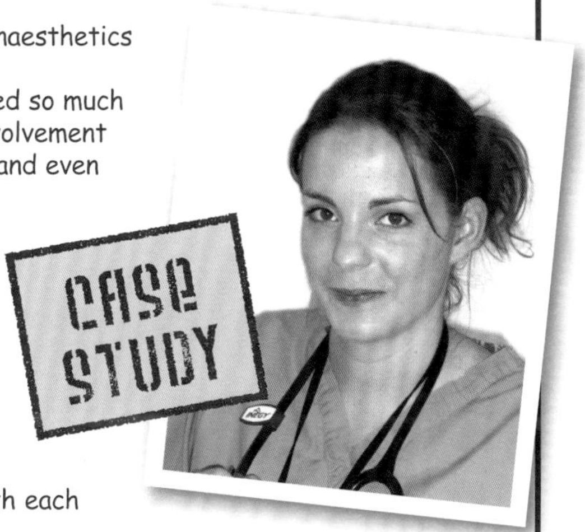

 I thought that an F1 post in anaesthetics would just give me insight into anaesthetics, but it actually offered so much more: working in intensive care, involvement in theatre lists, acute pain rounds and even outreach teams and crash teams.

The job required that I learned new practical skills every day (under expert tuition), and it really gave me an opportunity to develop my pharmacology and physiology knowledge. From recognising seriously ill patients to intubating patients crashing in resus, my confidence increased with each acute care situation.

CASE STUDY

I can now cannulate even the most difficult patient, insert central and arterial lines and manage patient airways from a simple chin lift to a double lumen tube intubation.

The acute care skills I developed in this post have been invaluable in my other jobs. So, if you aren't put off by the early starts, then I would recommend an anaesthetic job to any F1.

Dr Jennie Lambert
F1 Doctor
St. James Hospital, Leeds

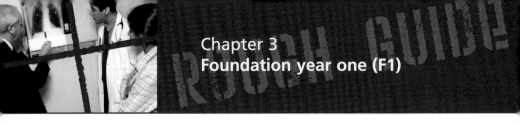
Your study time

Your foundation training programme director (FTPD) will ensure that you have access to a formal taught programme of education which addresses the professional elements of the *Curriculum.*

You will have up to three hours per week of protected, bleep-free time set aside for a timetabled learning programme. Alternatively, this time may be aggregated to give you seven days of whole day release.

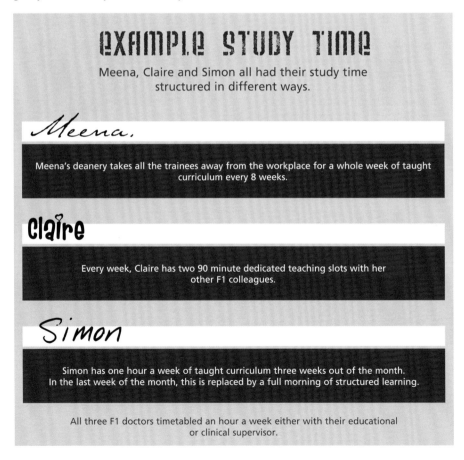

EXAMPLE STUDY TIME

Meena, Claire and Simon all had their study time structured in different ways.

Meena.

Meena's deanery takes all the trainees away from the workplace for a whole week of taught curriculum every 8 weeks.

Claire

Every week, Claire has two 90 minute dedicated teaching slots with her other F1 colleagues.

Simon

Simon has one hour a week of taught curriculum three weeks out of the month. In the last week of the month, this is replaced by a full morning of structured learning.

All three F1 doctors timetabled an hour a week either with their educational or clinical supervisor.

Assessment

Workplace-based assessment and feedback are central to the philosophy of foundation training. Regular assessment ensures you are progressing, provides documentary evidence of your achievements and can be used to identify any problems you are having early on.

Why am I being assessed?

1. **Public accountability.** Patients need assurance that all doctors have demonstrated their ability to practise in accordance with standards set out in publications such as the GMC's *Good Medical Practice*. You need to demonstrate that your overall performance is satisfactory before your postgraduate dean or foundation school director can recommended you to the GMC for full registration.

2. **Personal development.** Choosing a career in medicine means you've chosen a career where you can look forward to life-long learning. Workplace-based assessments provide you with constructive feedback that can inform and strengthen your personal development plans.

The goal is to help you provide better care to patients; and to help you strengthen any areas of weakness that are identified.

You will be assessed against the standard of competence that is expected of a doctor completing the F1 year. This means that, in your first days as a foundation doctor, you may not reach the standard required. Don't worry, this is to be expected and is NOT a failure. The assessments are designed to measure your progress through the year. At the end of F1, you will be expected to have progressed to a satisfactory level.

How and where will I be assessed?

Your assessments will be done in your workplace. Your educational supervisor wants to see what you actually do on the job and your ability to translate what you've learned into practice.

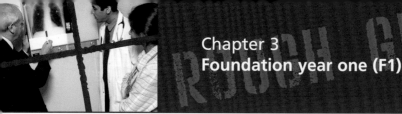
There are three types of assessment commonly used:

- **Multi-Source Feedback (MSF)** provides an opportunity for a number of your colleagues to rate your abilities and offer comments. The three tools currently in use are:

  o Mini Peer Assessment Tool (mini-PAT),

  o Team Assessment of Behaviours (TAB)

  o Multi-source feedback tool (used in Scotland).

  With all of these tools, you will be asked to submit a list of colleagues (including non-clinical members of your healthcare team) as possible raters/assessors. An administrator will contact these raters and will compile the results once sufficient responses are received. The report is sent to your educational supervisor, who will discuss the results and comments with you.

- **Direct observation of doctor/patient encounters** are observed clinical interactions which provide the opportunity for immediate feedback to the junior doctor. The two most commonly used tools are:

  o Direct Observation of Procedural Skills (DOPS)

  o Mini Clinical Evaluation Exercise (Mini-CEX).

EXAMPLE ASSESSMENT

Claire

Claire has a DOPS (direct observation of procedural skills) assessment in her first placement. She's only in her second month of the Foundation Programme and has elected to have an assessment on giving an intravenous injection to an elderly patient. She struggles to find a vein, but finally succeeds on the 3rd attempt. The results of her assessment show that she is 'below expectation' for a doctor who has completed her F1 year. This is as expected. She hasn't had much practise and still has 10 months to go before she's completed her F1 year. However she receives good feedback from her assessor on improvements she could make to her technique. On reassessment a month later, having practised the skill, she is seen to be competent.

During your placements, you should ask experienced colleagues (including SpRs, consultants, GP principals, plus experienced nurses and allied health professionals in the case of DOPS) to observe you performing particular procedure (DOPS) or clinical consultation (mini-CEX), rate your level of competence and provide feedback. It is your responsibility to arrange the assessments and submit copies of the reports.

- **Case-Based Discussion (CBD)** – this is a structured review of cases you have been involved in. It allows you to discuss your decision-making and clinical reasoning in a safe, non-judgemental environment with a senior clinician.

The assessments may sound intimidating, but they all come with instructions and training material for you and the assessors.

How will it all work?

The assessment tools used will vary, depending on your foundation school. At induction, your foundation school will provide you with details of exactly what assessments you are expected to complete, how many are required, when you should complete them and how to submit the results.

Your responsibilities

You are responsible for organising your own assessments. They typically take no more than one hour a month. You will need to find suitable cases and ask experienced colleagues to assess you. Do not leave your assessments until your final placement – your colleagues will not have time to complete all of the assessments in the last few weeks of the year; and you will not be popular.

All completed assessments should be kept in your portfolio, whatever the outcome. The idea is that you should improve from assessment to assessment. Your educational supervisor will need to review your portfolio at regular intervals during each foundation year.

TV07453

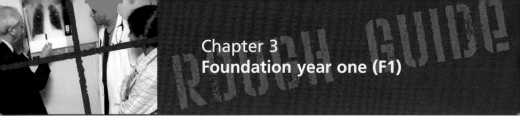

What do I get out of all this?

Put simply, you learn more. The assessments give you an opportunity to regularly receive direct and instant feedback from experienced members of staff.

The strengths and areas for development that are identified in the assessments will help you with your personal development planning for the next year.

The assessments will also inform your educational supervisor's report to the deanery at the end of F1. This is important to ensure you're recommended for full GMC registration at the end of F1.

What do I do if I have a problem or question?

Although you are responsible for your own assessments, there is plenty of help available. Talk to your educational supervisor first, or go to your foundation school website. You can also speak to your local administrator or Foundation Training Programme Director or Tutor (FTPD or FTPT).

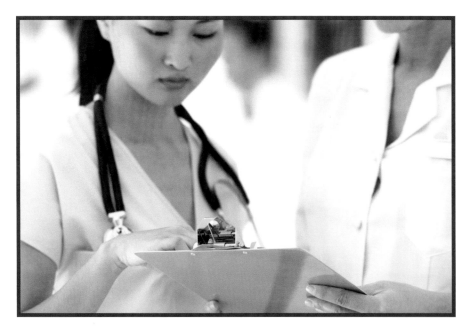

CASE STUDY

" Finding time to fill out assessment forms with my senior colleagues was quite difficult at the start of my placement. I was too focused on getting that perfect case where I could perform really well. I later realised that the idea of the assessments was not to score brilliantly throughout but to show the progression during the year.

Having the assessments and receiving feedback helped me improve my practice – it's definitely better to complete some assessments early on.

Keeping this in mind I made sure I kept the assessment forms close to hand. I've found that whilst I'm on call is the best time to pick up cases. Being able to follow a case you've admitted all the way through to discharge gives you a complete overview.

Case-based discussion gives you a good opportunity to raise concerns with your consultant. I had admitted an elderly lady with ascites and chronic renal failure who was suffering from dehydration. In trying to rehydrate her, she received too much fluid and slipped into pulmonary oedema. I felt guilty and thought I had given her poor treatment. Being able to discuss this case with my consultant reassured me that I had managed the case appropriately and improved my knowledge on the subject for the future. "

Dr Liam Sullivan

F1 Doctor
Manchester

EXAMPLE ASSESSMENT

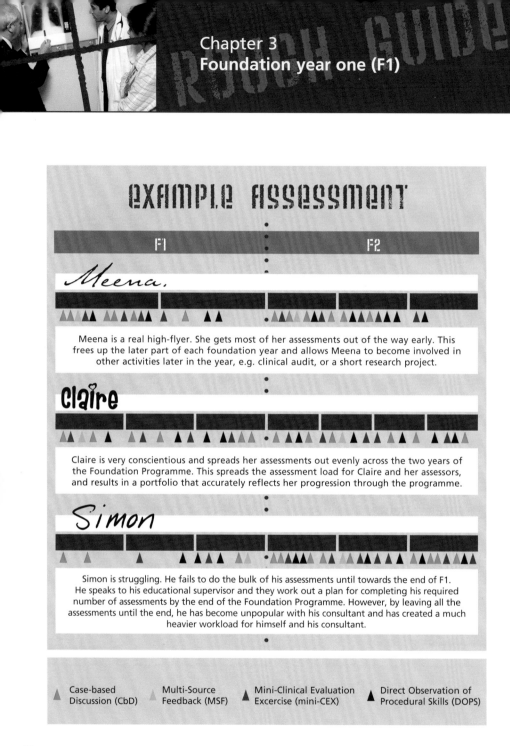

| F1 | F2 |

Meena.

Meena is a real high-flyer. She gets most of her assessments out of the way early. This frees up the later part of each foundation year and allows Meena to become involved in other activities later in the year, e.g. clinical audit, or a short research project.

Claire

Claire is very conscientious and spreads her assessments out evenly across the two years of the Foundation Programme. This spreads the assessment load for Claire and her assessors, and results in a portfolio that accurately reflects her progression through the programme.

Simon

Simon is struggling. He fails to do the bulk of his assessments until towards the end of F1. He speaks to his educational supervisor and they work out a plan for completing his required number of assessments by the end of the Foundation Programme. However, by leaving all the assessments until the end, he has become unpopular with his consultant and has created a much heavier workload for himself and his consultant.

▲ Case-based Discussion (CbD)   ▲ Multi-Source Feedback (MSF)   ▲ Mini-Clinical Evaluation Exercise (mini-CEX)   ▲ Direct Observation of Procedural Skills (DOPS)

Your Foundation Learning Portfolio

Your portfolio contains everything you need to manage your placements and monitor your progress on the Foundation Programme. Many foundation schools are using electronic portfolios where everything you do, all your assessments, etc will be kept online. However, if you are using a paper-based portfolio, keep it safe.

What's in the Foundation Learning Portfolio?

- list of competences required to successfully complete the foundation programme

- example forms to record meetings with your educational supervisor reflective practice and self appraisal

- educational agreement

- assessment forms

- personal development plan (PDP) including career planning

The portfolio will become your record of achievements throughout your foundation training. It is your responsibility to keep it up to date. Without it you will not be able to complete the Foundation Programme. You will have to submit your portfolio at the end of each year to show that you have reached the required level of competence to progress.

The Foundation Learning Portfolio is just the start. You will go on to gather evidence of your professional development and continue your education throughout your career.

An explanation of how to fill out your portfolio will accompany it, but on the next few pages we provide some pointers for two of the most important elements: assessments and your personal development plan.

YOUR PORTFOLIO SHOULD:

- Provide evidence of learning and achievement – both personal and professional
- Incorporate a record of descriptive and reflective learning and activity
- Support reflective practice

CASE STUDY

" I would recommend that all foundation doctors familiarise themselves with the Foundation Learning Portfolio as early as possible. It really is a useful tool and you will get out of the portfolio at least what you put into it.

Reflective practice, for example, helped me rationalise horrendous days, congratulate myself on jobs well done and chart my future practice. Although I have chosen my intended career, the prompts within the portfolio helped me to crystallise my ideas and plan my journey. The personal development plan helped me focus on my aims, expectations and learning needs prior to each post and to monitor my progress throughout the posts. I could therefore ask directly for the help I needed.

In addition to maintaining a record of my assessments, the Foundation Learning Portfolio provided the inspiration for me to include extras that are tailored to my intended career. I have added in details of my publications, presentations and conferences and courses I have attended, as well as teaching diaries to provide further evidence of my experiences. "

Dr Elizabeth Cotterell

F1 Doctor
University Hospital of North Staffordshire, Stoke-on-Trent

YOUR PORTFOLIO WILL:

- Record the range of experience, learning, education, training and assessment undertaken
- Allow for review of clinical practice on a regular basis and identify goals and competencies to be achieved
- Hold a learning agreement and documentation relating to appraisal and a personal development plan including career planning

Using assessments to develop your portfolio

This section will take you through the principles described by the GMC in *Good Medical Practice*. Each competence is listed down the left side and a recommended approach to its assessment is listed down the right side. You can choose how you want to demonstrate that you have achieved a competence, so this list should only be used as a guide.

1. Good Clinical Care

Competence	Assessment tools
1.1 Demonstrates the knowledge, attitudes, behaviours, skills and competences to be able to take a history and examine patients, prescribe safely and keep an accurate and relevant medical record	
i) History taking	Mini-CEX/CbD
ii) Examination	Mini-CEX/CbD
iii) Diagnosis and clinical decision-making	Mini-CEX/CbD
iv) Safe prescribing	CbD
v) Medical record-keeping, letters etc	CbD
1.2 Demonstrates appropriate time management and organisational decision-making	**MSF/CbD**

1. Good Clinical Care (cont.)

Competence	Assessment tools
1.3 Understands and applies the basis of maintaining good quality care and ensuring and promoting patient safety	
i) The patient as the centre of care	Mini-CEX/CbD/MSF
ii) Makes patient safety a priority in own clinical practice.	CbD/MSF
iii) Understands the importance of good team-working for patient safety	CbD/MSF
iv) Understands the principles of quality and safety improvement	CbD/MSF
v) Understands the needs of patients who have been subject to medical harm or errors	CbD
1.4 Demonstrates the knowledge, skills, attitudes and behaviours to reduce the risk of cross-infection	**DOPS/Mini-CEX/MSF**
1.5 Understands that clinical governance is the over-arching framework that unites a range of quality improvement activities. This safeguards high standards of care and facilitates the development of improved clinical services	**CbD**
1.6 Demonstrates the knowledge, skills, attitudes and behaviours to ensure basic nutritional care	**Mini-CEX/CbD**
1.7 Demonstrates the knowledge, skills, attitudes and behaviours to be able to educate patients effectively	

1. Good Clinical Care (cont.)

Competence	Assessment tools
(i) Educating patients about disease prevention, investigations and therapy	Mini-CEX/CbD
(ii) Environmental, biological and lifestyle risk factors	Mini-CEX/CbD
(iii) Smoking	Mini-CEX/CbD
(iv) Alcohol	Mini-CEX/CbD
(v) Epidemiology and screening	Mini-CEX/CbD
1.8 Demonstrates the knowledge and skills to cope with ethical and legal issues which occur during the management of patients with general medical problems	
(i) Medical ethical principles and confidentiality	CbD/MSF
(ii) Valid consent	CbD/DOPS
(iii) Legal framework of medical practice	CbD

2. Maintaining good medical practice

Competence	Assessment tools
2.1 Demonstrates the knowledge, attitudes, behaviours, skills and competences needed to start self-directed life-long learning	MSF/Use of portfolio/ Educational and clinical supervisor's report
2.2 Demonstrates knowledge, skills, attitudes and behaviours to use evidence and guidelines that will benefit patient care	MSF/CbD
2.3 Demonstrates the knowledge, skills, attitudes and behaviours to use audit to improve patient care	Involvement in audit (report should be included in Foundation Learning Portfolio)

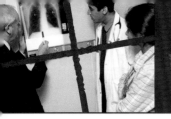

3. Teaching and Training

Competence	Assessment tools
Demonstrates the knowledge, skills, attitudes and behaviours to undertake a teaching role	
(i) Teaching	MSF
(ii) Presentations	MSF/Supervisor's report

4. Relationship with patients and communications skills

Competence	Assessment tools
Demonstrates the knowledge, skills, attitudes and behaviours to be able to communicate effectively with patients, relatives and colleagues in the circumstances outlined below	
(i) Within a consultation	Mini-CEX/MSF
(ii) Breaking bad news	Mini-CEX/MSF
(iii) Complaints	Mini-CEX/CbD/MSF

5. Working with colleagues

Competence	Assessment tools
Demonstrates effective teamwork skills within the clinical team and in the larger medical context	
(i) Communication with colleagues and teamwork	MSF
(ii) Interface with different specialties, and with other professionals, including: members of a team, clinical team and support services, hospital and GP, hospital and other agencies, e.g. social services, police	CbD
(iii) Relevance of outside bodies	CbD

6. Professional Behaviour and Probity

Competence	Assessment tools
Develops the knowledge, skills, attitudes and behaviours to always act in a professional manner	
(i) Doctor-patient relationships	Mini-CEX/DOPS/CbD/MSF
(ii) Health and handling stress	MSF

7. Acute Care

Competence	Assessment tools
7.1 Core skills in relation to acute illness	
i) Promptly assesses the acutely ill or collapsed patient	Mini-CEX/CbD
ii) Identifies and responds to acutely abnormal physiology	Mini-CEX/CbD
iii) Where appropriate, delivers a fluid challenge safely to an acutely ill patient	Mini-CEX/DOPS
iv) Reassesses ill patients appropriately after initiation of treatment	Mini-CEX/CbD
v) Requests senior or more experienced help when appropriate	Mini-CEX/MSF
vi) Undertakes a secondary survey to establish differential diagnosis	Mini-CEX/CbD
vii) Obtains an arterial blood gas sample safely, interprets results correctly	DOPS
viii) Manages patients with impaired consciousness including convulsions	Mini-CEX/CbD
ix) uses common analgesic drugs safely and effectively	Mini-CEX/CbD
x) Understands and applies the principles of managing a patient following self-harm	Mini-CEX/CbD
xi) Understands and applies the principles of managing a patient with an acute confusional state or psychosis	Mini-CEX/CbD
xii) Ensures safe continuing care of patients on handover between shifts, on call staff or with "hospital at night" team by meticulous attention to detail and reflection on performance	CbD/MSF

7. Acute Care (cont.)

Competence	Assessment tools
xiii) Considers appropriateness of interventions according to patients' wishes, severity of illness and chronic or co-morbid diseases	Mini-CEX/CbD
7.2 Demonstrates the knowledge, competences and skills to be able to recognise critically ill patients, take part in advanced life support, feel confident to initiate resuscitation, lead the team where necessary and use the local protocol for deciding when not to resuscitate patients	
(i) Resuscitation	Certificates of Completion of Intermediate Life Support Course (or equivalent), Advanced Life Support (or equivalent) Mini-CEX
ii) Discusses Do Not Attempt Resuscitation (DNAR) orders/advance directives appropriately	Mini-CEX/CbD
7.3 Demonstrates the knowledge, competences and skills to be able to function safely in an acute 'take' team	**CbD/MSF**
7.4 Demonstrates the knowledge and skills to be able to plan discharge for patients, starting from the point of admission and taking into account the effects of any chronic disease	**CbD/MSF**
7.5 Demonstrates the knowledge and skills to be able to select, appropriately request and accurately interpret reports of the frequently used investigations listed below. For all investigations it is vital that foundation doctors recognise abnormalities which need immediate action	

7. Acute Care (cont.)

Competence	Assessment tools
(i) Full blood count Urea and electrolytes Blood glucose Cardiac markers Liver function tests Amylase Calcium and phosphate Coagulation studies Arterial blood gases Inflammatory markers	CbD/Mini-CEX
(ii) 12 lead ECG	CbD/DOPS
(iii) Peak flow, spirometry	CbD/DOPS
(iv) Chest X-ray Abdominal X-ray Trauma radiography Ultrasound, CT and MRI	CbD/Mini-CEX
(v) Microbiological samples	CbD

8. Practical Procedures

Competence	Assessment tools
F1 Procedures that F1 doctors should be competent and confident to do and teach to undergraduates:	
• venepuncture and IV cannulation • local anaesthetics • arterial puncture in an adult • blood cultures from peripheral and central sites • subcutaneous, intradermal, intramuscular and intravenous injections • IV medications • intravenous infusions, including the prescription of fluids, blood and blood products • ECG • spirometry and peak flow • urethral catheterisation • airway care, including simple adjuncts • nasogastric tube insertion.	DOPS
During F2, doctors are expected to maintain and improve their skills in the above procedures. By the end of the year they should be able to help others with difficult procedures and guide F1 doctors in teaching others. **Foundation doctors will be able to extend the range of procedures they can do. Each specialty will specify an appropriate range of procedures in which foundation doctors will be expected to become proficient, e.g.**	
• aspiration of pleural fluid or air • skin suturing • lumbar puncture • insertion of a central venous pressure line • aspiration of joint effusion.	DOPS

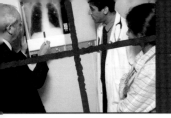
EXAMPLE EVIDENCE GATHERING

Meena, Claire and Simon want to gather evidence for the following competence:

**Understands and applies the principle of managing a
patient following self harm.**

Meena.

Meena uses a case for a case-based discussion (CbD) with her educational supervisor. She brings
out all the above points and also demonstrates in the discussion that she understands:
- Psychological causes requiring social services or police intervention
- How to access Toxbase if appropriate
- Knowledge of child protection concerns

Claire

Claire writes a short reflective document following admission of a patient who took
an overdose of tablets. The reflection indicates that she understands the principles of
managing a patient following self harm. She then includes this in her portfolio.

Simon

Simon asks to be observed as a mini-CEX when taking the history,
so that he can demonstrate the following skills in his history taking:
- Taking a focused history
- Demonstrating tolerance and understanding

Simon and Meena gain the competences using the suggested assessment tools, but Claire has taken
the opportunity to reflect to show her understanding of the competence. Each of the foundation
doctors is able to demonstrate their competence in this core skill using different assessment tools.

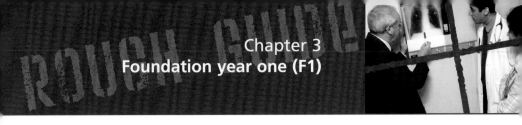

How to get the best out of your Personal Development Plan (PDP)

Within the Foundation Learning Portfolio is a section for your very own personal development plan. This will help you think about what educational experiences you'd like to have in the coming months.

Putting this together need not be a daunting task if you follow a few simple guidelines. Keep your PDP:

- **Simple** – particularly in year one as it is an evolving process
- **Work-based** – focus on the job you are doing
- **Achievable** – set yourself realistic goals and timeframes
- **Relevant** – both to you and your patients.

Getting started

The structure and content of PDPs will vary depending on your learning needs.
All PDPs address a common set of questions:

- What are my learning needs?
- How do I identify these needs?
- How and when will I address these learning needs?
- How do I show my learning needs have been met?

Finding out what you don't know can be tough, but your first port of call should be the *Curriculum*. This will clue you into the knowledge, skills and attitudes required to complete the Foundation Programme.

You and your educational supervisor can discuss exactly which elements would be

Example personal development plan form

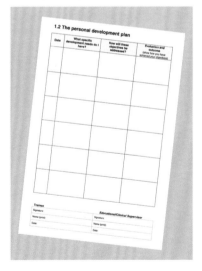

appropriate to work on in each placement. You should not be constrained by the *Curriculum* as the benefit of a PDP is that it allows you to develop in areas that are outside of the *Curriculum*. It may be that you also want to undertake 'taster' sessions in clinical areas you do not have a full placement in and this can be incorporated within your PDP.

Assessment
Multi-Source Feedback

CASE STUDY

"The multi-source feedback assessment tool we used was the Mini Peer Assessment Tool (mini PAT), which I found very useful. When starting work, fellow colleagues sometimes commend your actions. Occasionally a senior will be impressed and mention it to you. Rarely, however, does anyone write it down, which is one of the reasons this tool is so valuable.

How it works:

"Each foundation doctor is responsible for nominating their assessors. These may include any member of the team from consultants to F1s, sisters and allied healthcare professionals. They each receive a questionnaire covering many aspects of your performance from medical knowledge to professional attitude. Once completed, they are sent anonymously to a central office. You also complete the questionnaire and the results are collected to present your self-appraisal ratings against your chosen assessor's ratings and the national average. Individual comments can be added in the questionnaire and are listed with your results.

The results

"It can be disconcerting reading criticism, no matter how constructive. In my mini PAT, I received a comment that I could improve my practice by discussing clinical management with my seniors more frequently. I had felt that I didn't want to bother my seniors with minor management issues and the feedback has helped me realise that this can often benefit the team and patient care.

Top tips

"Plan which placement you'll be completing the assessment in ahead of time, make sure that you choose the maximum of assessors possible, and finally don't forget the harshest assessors are often your friends."

Dr Liam Sullivan
F1 Doctor
Manchester

Q-PORTFOLIOS
by Dr Jennie Lambert, F1 Doctor

An e-portfolio is a great way to store all your achievements over the Foundation Programme and is a useful tool for both your end of year RITAs and your application to specialty training. Some foundation schools are using the NHS e-portfolio as a compulsory part of your in job assessment. If so, you will receive a user name and password from your school. If not, the BMA and doctors.net both offer good alternatives.

PDP

At the start of your F1 year, you will need to develop a Personal Development Plan (PDP) in your portfolio. This enables you to focus your learning over the year. My advice is to work through the Foundation Programme Curriculum and pick out areas you wish to work on. Record what you are going to do to develop this area, how you will know you have achieved it and how long this should take.

Presented Evidence

The portfolio offers you the chance to record 'presented evidence'. This includes:

- lectures, tutorials, courses and exams you have attended;
- recording procedures you have assisted with or completed;
- reflective practice to record experiences and what you have learnt from them;
- a place to note reading you have done and
- a place to show presentations you have given.

These sections are worth completing as you go through the year to give you a record of, and show your commitment to, teaching and learning. This will help you to gain your full GMC registration and aid your next job applications.

Technical advice
- Click on "add new" at the bottom of the presented evidence page to add new evidence.

Top Tips!

Your portfolio should be...
- Personal
- Clear
- Structured

Your portfolio should...
- Provide evidence of progress and development
- Show achievements
- Demonstrate reflection

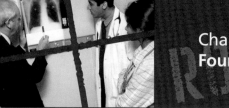
- If using the NHS e-portfolio, you need to add your entry to your "shared portfolio" when the submission is complete. Then you must sign your log prior to your next educational supervisor meeting to allow them to see your work.

Careers Management

The careers management section of the e-portfolio allows you to keep a log of all the research you do and opportunities you take to find your ideal specialty. This gives you a chance to keep on track of your career planning and gives you evidence to support your commitment to a certain career. It will help with applications and interviews.

Technical advice

- You simply add an entry for each time you do something/read something career related.

Assessments

The assessment section of the e-portfolio gives you a chance to print off a guide for your assessors on how to fill in the assessments, an opportunity to see blank forms so you know what you are being assessed on and enables you to see completed assessments. If you are finding it hard to get a senior colleague to sit down by a computer to do your assessments I would recommend printing off a blank sheet and carrying it around with you until they have spare time to complete it. They can then fill in the form away from the computer and put the information in later at a more convenient time (this is especially helpful with surgeons, however, you will need to keep checking your e-portfolio to make sure they have submitted the assessment).

Evidence Log

The evidence log facility allows you to save the current screen page in front of you into an evidence log folder. You can then associate this page with parts of the Foundation Programme Curriculum to demonstrate that you are reaching these outcomes.

For example, if you used DOPS to demonstrate that you can take and interpret an arterial blood gas, you can save your DOPS page in the evidence log and associate it electronically with the part of the curriculum that it relates to.

This is especially useful to do in preparation for your RITA.

Technical advice
- At the bottom of any e-portfolio page, you can click on 'add this page to your evidence log'
- In your RITA, all you need to do is click on 'evidence log' in the menu column and you can demonstrate all your activities and how you are meeting the curricula outcomes on one simple page.

The NHS e-portfolio is always being updated, so keep checking the site to make sure you are using all the areas of the e-portfolio available to you. I would also suggest that you print out key sections such as your PDP, assessments and supervisor reports as well as any hard work you have done on the above sections as a paper portfolio as a back up.

Another top tip is to make sure you log off. On the communal hospital computers if you have not logged out, even if you close the browser, the next person to go to the site automatically logs on to your page and could therefore alter any of your submissions.

The NHS e-portfolios can be found at www.nhseportfolios.org.

Your PDP is not just about foundation competences, but how you develop as a doctor. Reflective practice should be a large part of this. As you fill in each section of the PDP, spend some time reviewing the content of that section to understand:

- What lessons can be learned?
- What are the implications for you, your patients and the wider healthcare team?
- Can you identify skills and knowledge gaps?
- How can you best develop a particular area?

Your PDP should include a personal account of the experiences you have had and your reflections on them. It doesn't all need to be shared with your supervisor.

The reflective practice form in your portfolio will help you focus you on how experiences or events affect you, the patient and the healthcare team. Reflective practice also encourages you to think about how things might be done differently.

Your educational supervisor will be happy to help you in the construction of this element of the portfolio but it is essentially your document, your plan and your future.

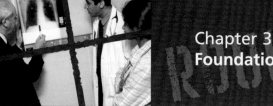

Becoming a fully registered doctor

After satisfactorily completing 12 months of training in F1 posts and demonstrating that you have achieved the required competences you are eligible for full registration with the GMC. It's important to remember that your assessments and Foundation Learning Portfolio will help your university/postgraduate dean to recommend you for full registration.

Applying for full registration

a. **Complete an application form** – download a full registration application form from the GMC website and fill in the first page with your personal details. Leave the second page (Certificate of Experience) blank.

b. **Organise a Certificate of Experience** – forward the Certificate of Experience document to your medical school or postgraduate dean - they will need to complete the document and return it to you. Remember to include Certificates of Satisfactory Service (which you will receive at the end of each post) when submitting the request.

c. **Forward your application to the GMC** – Once you have received your completed Certificate of Experience, attach it to your application form, remembering to include the £290 registration fee, and send it to the GMC.

Within five working days, the GMC will be in contact to acknowledge receipt of your application. Once registration has been granted, a certificate confirming your registration will be sent to you.

You will then be able to continue your medical education and training as a fully registered doctor.

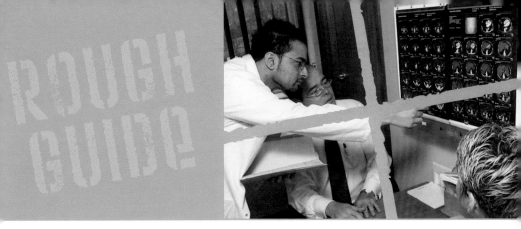

ROUGH GUIDE

Chapter 4
Foundation year two (F2)

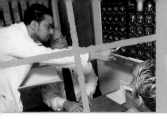
The placements

The Foundation Programme is designed to give you the opportunity to access a wide range of specialty placements. The placements you can undertake will depend on how F2 allocations are made in your foundation school. Placements will be combined carefully to provide you with the ability to gain the required F2 competences.

Placements in F2 usually consist of three 4-month specialty placements. You may also have the opportunity to have embedded 'tasters', where you work for a week in another specialty. Your educational supervisor will arrange this with you.

By expressing your preferred specialties (either at application or during your first year rotation), you will have some choice in the rotation that you get in the second foundation year.

However, not everyone will get the specialties they request. There are a finite number of available jobs in any one specialty.

Don't worry though, your F2 placement choices will not have a direct bearing on your chances of getting into your specialty training programme of choice at the end of the Foundation Programme. Foundation training is about achieving the generic skills needed by all doctors in any area of practice.

New placements available to trainees:

• General practice

• Shortage specialties (e.g. those specialties in which there has not traditionally been access in the early postgraduate years)

• Academic medicine

About general practice placements

By the time you enter the second foundation year all of your clinical experience as a doctor will have been in a secondary care setting. A placement in general practice will provide an opportunity for you to care for patients in a very different environment: their own communities.

This is typically where illness is first seen and it is where your patients return after recovery. This placement will allow you to follow your patient through the entire patient experience, from the presentation of acute illness, through investigation, diagnosis and management to recovery or rehabilitation. This will improve your understanding of your patients and enable you to provide better care.

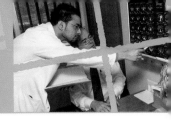

Throughout the attachment you will be encouraged to consider and reflect on the impact on your patient of the hospital environment, the general practice environment, and the interface between the two. What does it feel like to be taken ill and then taken away from home and family to hospital?

The manner of presentation of acutely ill patients is different in general practice and illnesses are seen at a much earlier stage in their development. Their management at this stage requires different skills both in clinical method and risk assessment. Learning about this aspect of patient care will give you a greater understanding of your patients.

You will have an opportunity to explore the consultation as a behavioural interaction between doctor and patient and to rehearse the skills that lead to better outcomes for all involved.

The nuts and bolts of a general practice placement

There will be an initial induction, working with the GPs and members of the extended primary care team. Patterns of team working are often different in primary care; teams tend to work in a multidisciplinary fashion on a smaller organisational scale. Later in the attachment you will have the opportunity to see patients under appropriate supervision both in the surgery and potentially, in their own homes.

A trained supervisor will be working with you to ensure that you gain all you can from the learning opportunities presented. You should expect to spend (on average) about six half-days per week seeing patients, working with GPs and other team members. You will spend the rest of the time on project work, work-based teaching, assessments and attending teaching sessions in the foundation school.

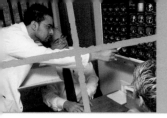

About shortage specialties

There are a number of specialties that are actively recruiting and some have developed extremely innovative training programmes. There are opportunities to experience these specialties much earlier in your postgraduate medical education than ever before. These specialties include:

- audiological medicine
- chemical pathology/metabolic medicine
- clinical genetics
- genito-urinary medicine
- intensive care medicine/critical care medicine
- medical microbiology
- nuclear medicine
- psychiatry
- public health medicine
- virology
- allergy
- histopathology
- immunology
- radiology

The availability of these placements and others will depend on which programme you are in.

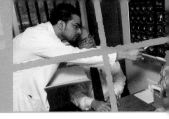

About academic placements

If you fancy yourself as the person who finds a cure for cancer and are considering a career in research, or you would like to share your knowledge and go into education, an academic clinical attachment will give you first hand experience of this environment.

You can combine research and project work with your clinical attachment so you can gain all the foundation competences and also develop your research skills.

The nuts and bolts of an academic placement

There are two ways you can experience the academic life. Firstly, you can apply for a fully integrated one or two-year clinical and research placement based in a single department. This will enable you to more fully participate in the workings of the academic department and better develop your research skills, while seeing patients and achieving the educational goals common to all Foundation Programme trainees.

Alternatively, if you would rather experience just a taster of the academic environment, you can apply for a four-month attachment to an academic department.

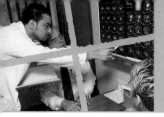
Study leave

In F2, you are eligible for 30 days study leave per year. A minimum of 10 days of your study leave will be used for a formal educational programme in generic professional training and other aspects of F2 training.

Less than full-time trainees are eligible for study leave calculated pro rata based on their training commitments.

Study leave is for providing education and training not easily achieved in the clinical setting. It will not be needed to support specialist examinations. Specialist exams are changing and new methods of selection into specialty training are being developed.

You should plan your study leave as far in advance as possible. It is an integral part of your education and training. Your educational supervisor will work with you to decide how your leave can be used most effectively.

What to do with your study leave

At least 10 days per year of your study leave will be used to support the learning objectives of the required formal education programme in generic professional training.

This could include:

- participation in interactive sessions and attending formally arranged activities such as presentations from outside speakers
- simulation programmes
- advanced life support (ALS) training
- undertaking a clinical audit project within an interprofessional action learning team.

You can use the remaining time and funding to learn about different clinical specialties. For example, you could do experiential placements on special interest or embedded 'taster' programmes. This gives you the chance to explore different career opportunities as well as to develop an understanding of how the specialty contributes to patient care.

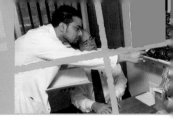

Assessment

You will be assessed in F2 using the same methods as in the F1 year and you will be assessed to the standard of competence that an F2 doctor should have attained at the end of their F2 year. All the information you need will be in the Foundation Learning Portfolio you will have received during your F1 induction.

Your assessments will be used by your postgraduate dean to decide whether or not you can be signed up as having satisfactorily completed the programme. The assessments are therefore used to make important decisions about progress and provide formative feedback along the way.

Once you have completed all the assessments satisfactorily, you will receive a Foundation Achievement of Competency Document (FACD). After this, your foundation training is complete.

Your Foundation Learning Portfolio

In addition to adding your completed assessments to the portfolio, you will continue to build your portfolio throughout F2. This will include:

- personal development plan
- educational agreements
- records of meetings with your educational supervisor
- reflective practice.

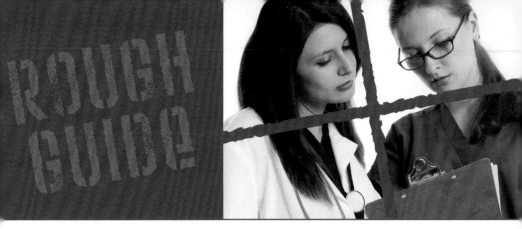

Chapter 5
Life after
foundation training

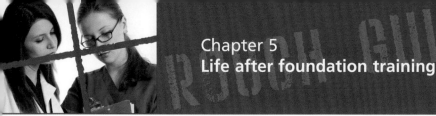

Towards the end of your foundation training, you will compete for entry directly into specialty registrar (StR) training for either general practice or hospital-based specialties. You will also have the opportunity to compete for a place on a combined academic clinical training programme if you wish.

Recruitment and selection into specialty training will commence about half-way through the second year of foundation training and you need to make your decisions about which career path to follow before applying.

Advice and support in planning your career is available throughout foundation training. This advice will seek to align your aptitudes and aspirations with employment opportunities and future workforce requirements of the NHS. Don't wait until you are six months into your F2 year to start thinking about your career, though. Start now.

Specialty/GP training

PMETB and the medical royal colleges have been charged with developing new competence-based curricula covering all aspects of specialty training from the completion of foundation training through to acquisition of a Certificate of Completion of Training (CCT). They will also be reviewing the length of individual programmes to ensure doctors reach CCT in the optimum timescale.

The new curricula came into effect from August 2007 and will continue to be refined over the next few years.

The aim will be to provide organised, structured programmes with clear curricula, assessment and appraisal which integrates the former SHO and SpR training into a seamless "run-through" training programme.

Please check www.pmetb.org.uk, www.mmc.nhs.uk and the websites of the medical royal colleges for the latest information on the new specialty training programmes.

In the meantime...

You shouldn't wait until the last minute to think about your career. Start your research now and discuss your options with your clinical supervisors and the relevant medical royal college(s).

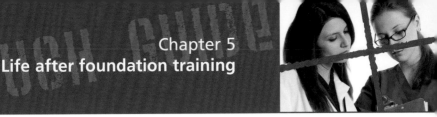

UK MMC Career Framework

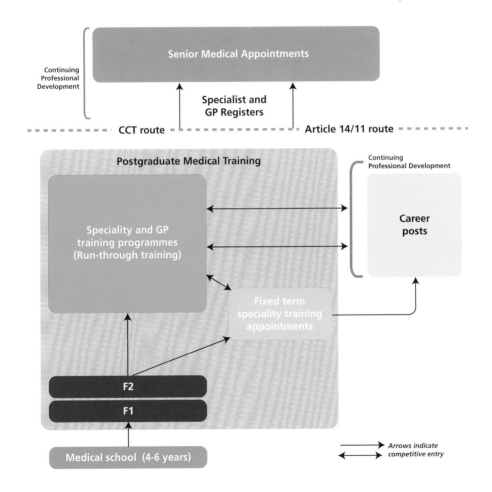

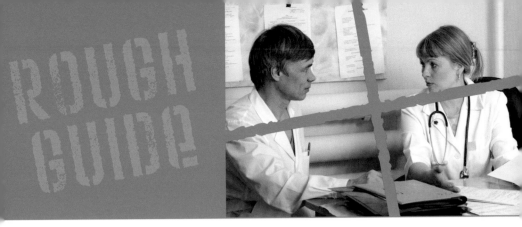

Chapter 6
Careers advice

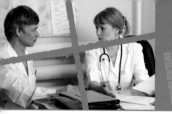

One of the aims of the Foundation Programme is to give you the opportunity to explore different career options. In addition to rotating through a range of specialties and healthcare settings, you will have access to information and advice about current and future career opportunities. Choosing which career path to follow needs a great deal of thought. Personal choice needs to be aligned with aptitude, strengths and interests as well as a realistic consideration of the extent of competition for and the availability of vacancies on training programmes.

As you plan your second year placements and prepare to refine your options for applying for specialty training programmes you might like to make use of some of the following resources:

Deanery/foundation school career advisors

The availability of good career advice is an underlying principle of Modernising Medical Careers. Each deanery or foundation school will therefore have career advisors who will offer personal and general career advice.

You

You are your best resource. Think about your own strengths, interests and aptitudes. Getting good career advice is not just about being spoon-fed information, it's about taking a critical and constructive look at yourself.

You should also bear in mind that competition in some specialties is immense. You need to think about the supply and demand of doctors for the career opportunities in front of you. For years, too many doctors have wanted careers in hospital specialties such as general medicine, general surgery and obstetrics and gynaecology, and not enough wanted careers in specialties like radiology, geriatrics and psychiatry.

During your Foundation Programme training you might like to:

- set up your own informal discussion groups about career progression
- use your learning portfolio as a tool to reflect on career development
- apply for taster experiences in specialties that you have not had a chance to experience in F1 or in F2 as full placements.

Clinical and educational supervisors

During the Foundation Programme, you will be working with a number of different doctors in a range of specialties. They will be able to give specialty-specific advice. Even if your supervisors are unable to answer all of your questions, they will be able to help you reflect on your strengths and weaknesses as you seek to determine which career options best match your emerging skills, aptitudes and attitudes.

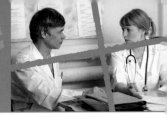

Career planning tools

Some deaneries are evaluating career planning tools like Sci59 or Myers Briggs which help you understand yourself better and can point you in the direction of a career that might suit you. These tools are seldom the 'answer' to planning a career in medicine but may be a useful place to start a discussion with peers, a supervisor or career advisor.

Occupational health

Occasionally, doctors have physical, emotional or psychological problems which might have an impact on their future career choice. If you need confidential help or support, you can refer yourself to your trust's occupational health service or access other support services through your postgraduate deanery.

The web

No list of resources is complete without a list of useful web links. Here are a few sites that could help you down the path of decisiveness.

NHS Medical Careers is a new website, launching in August 2007. It will support medical students and doctors in training as they plan their specialty careers. It is designed to provide a structured, organised way to think about choosing a specialty and uses a four-stage approach to career planning: *Understanding Yourself, Exploring Options, Choosing a Specialty* and *Getting into Training*. It combines interactive tools and some of the most in-depth information around all specialties in one place, for the first time. More information about this site in the run-up to its launch, will be available via www.nhsemployers.org and will also be linked from www.foundationprogramme.nhs.uk

BMJCareers (www.bmjcareers.com). In addition to job advertisements, BMJCareers provides information about career opportunities in medicine and related fields. The BMJ Careers Advice Zone also provides an interactive and impartial careers advice service which can be reached at www.bmjcareersadvicezone.synergynewmedia.co.uk.

Postgraduate deanery websites. Local deanery sites describe the specialty training opportunities available together with contact details for training programmes. Go to www.foundationprogramme.nhs.uk/deaneries for a full list of deaneries in the UK and links to their websites.

Medical royal college websites. The colleges are responsible for setting the standards for specialty training and provide information about current and future specialty training pathways, requirements and curricula.

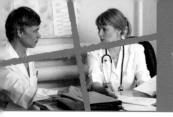

UK Foundation Programme Office (www.foundationprogramme.nhs.uk). This website has been developed as a central point of official information on the Foundation Programme for medical students, foundation doctors, and those involved in delivering the Foundation Programme across the UK. It contains copies of all the key documents required by the foundation programme and links to helpful websites, as well as discussion forums.

Postgraduate Medical Education and Training Board (www.pmetb.org.uk). The PMETB is the governing body which sets educational standards for postgraduate education from the F2 year and beyond.

Modernising Medical Careers (www.mmc.nhs.uk). In addition to providing news of latest developments in postgraduate medical education, the MMC website has a number of links to other useful career information resources.

DOS AND DON'TS FOR MANAGING YOUR CAREER

Dos	Don'ts
Do listen to and absorb the experiences of others more senior to you	Don't choose your future career on the basis of just one charismatic consultant or registrar's experience
Do seek out help that is available to help you think about your career options	Don't assume that others know what's best for you or expect others to tell you what to do
Do take a constructive view about other people's career experiences	Don't automatically be put off a particular career because of someone else's less positive experiences
Do be proactive about finding out the information and advice you need to begin to make a more informed choice about your career	Don't expect to be spoon-fed with careers information or advice
Do take every opportunity that is offered to you to help you look at your career development in more depth	Don't assume that sessions which look explicitly at careers in more depth will give you all the answers you require
Do view your career development as a life-long process that will require continual self-monitoring and review	Don't think that making your career choice is easy
Do think about your personality and skills, life experiences, ambitions and plans for the future.	Don't assume that you'll get it right on the first attempt.

Based on the Career Handbook for Medical Students, Binding, C and Anderson, D (Eds).

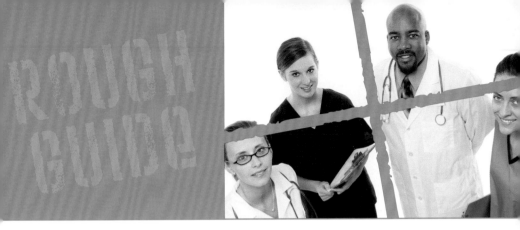

Chapter 7
What else?

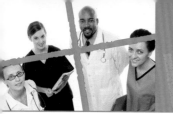

Obviously there's a lot more to say about the Foundation Programme, but we've gathered here some further information based on frequently asked questions.

Flexibility   53
   Trainees needing flexible training
   Deferring the start of the programme
   Out of phase trainees
   Time out of the Foundation Programme

Location   57
   Inter-deanery transfers
   Permanent withdrawal
   Gaining competences outside the UK

Trainees in difficulty   59
   What happens if things go wrong?

Who's who?   63
   Clinical supervisor
   Educational supervisor
   Foundation training programme director
   Clinical tutor
   Foundation schools
   Postgraduate deaneries
   Undergraduate dean/medical school
   General Medical Council
   Postgraduate Medical Education and Training Board
   Medical royal colleges
   UK Foundation Programme Office
   Healthcare organisation/employers

Further information   71
   Foundation Programme Curriculum
   Operational Framework for Foundation Training

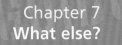
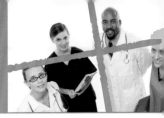

Flexibility

Trainees needing less than full-time training

If you wish to train flexibly, fair and equitable procedures will be in place to ensure that equal opportunities are available for you.

The criteria to allow trainees to access flexible training, as well as the funding and study leave arrangements will be explicit and fair. Currently, the main reasons for undertaking flexible training are:

- childcare
- disability or ill-health
- caring for an ill/disabled partner, relative or other dependant

Doctors wishing to train flexibly must compete for entry into foundation training on an equal basis with other applicants. You do not need to state your desire to train flexibly when you apply but we recommend that you discuss your intentions with the postgraduate deanery as soon as possible so your eligibility can be assessed.

You should formally declare your intention to train flexibly as soon as possible after you are informed of your acceptance to a foundation school in order to facilitate the process.

Doctors must undertake training on at least a half-time basis in order to comply with the requirements of the European Specialist Qualification Order (1995). In line with recent changes, arrangements for flexible training will usually be either:

- through reduced sessions within established full-time posts
- where a training slot is divided between two trainees, with additional sessional in-put from the deanery (in such a 'slot share' two flexible trainees share an educational post but not a contract and are employed and paid as individuals.)

Exceptionally, supernumerary flexible training will be considered where circumstances are such that this is the only way foundation training can be undertaken, for instance when a suitable partner cannot be found, or when flexible training is needed at short notice.

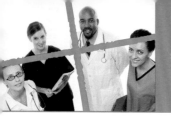
You must complete a total of two years whole time equivalence of foundation training before you receive an FACD, even if you achieved all the competences before the end of the two years.

If you are training flexibly, you are entitled to full financial access to the study leave allocation. Time for study leave should be calculated pro rata based on your hours of training.

Deferring the start of the programme

Once you have been accepted onto a two-year Foundation Programme, you may defer your start date with the agreement of your postgraduate dean or foundation school/training programme director. You must have good reasons to do this (e.g. in order to undertake a BSc) and it would usually be for one year only.

You will usually need to give at least three months notice of your intention to defer in order to allow your foundation placement to be filled by another trainee.

You cannot defer the start of stand-alone first year or second year appointments (i.e. not part of a two-year programme) except in exceptional circumstances (e.g. on the grounds of health).

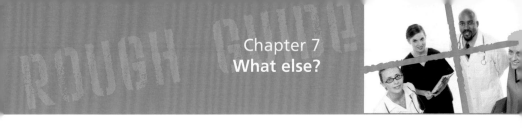
Out of phase trainees

Most medical graduates complete medical school training in July and anticipate starting foundation training in early August after graduation. The exception to this are those graduates who are out of phase because they attend medical schools with a planned graduation date other than July, which means that they do not start foundation training in August. This will be phased out in early 2008 when all subsequent medical graduates will commence foundation training in August.

However, medical schools that have late graduation dates will have plans in place with the postgraduate deanery to ensure the Foundation Programme placements are offered that start at a time that is compatible with your local graduation.

If you have secured a Foundation Programme post but can't start training in August (because of failure at finals or for personal reasons such as pregnancy) you must notify the postgraduate deanery as soon as possible.

If you know you can't start training at the normal time, you should make this clear on your application form. This will not influence the outcome of your application. If you fail finals, don't worry about your place on the Foundation Programme. You should advise the foundation school or deanery as soon as possible so that the start date of your foundation training can be reconsidered.

Time out of the programme

If you want to take time out of the programme, you should discuss it initially with your educational supervisor or foundation programme training director.

Although you are expected to complete your two-year programme as quickly as possible, it may be acceptable to take time out if you have good reasons, for example:

- for domestic reasons
- for health reasons
- for personal reasons
- to work elsewhere
- to travel

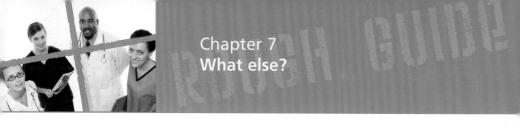
How to take time out

If you decide to take time out, you must complete a Time Out of Foundation Programme (TOFP) proforma, which you can get from your foundation training programme director (FTPD). This should be sent to the FTPD by the end of the sixth month of your first year in the programme unless there are extenuating circumstances such as health or other personal reasons.

Time out of the two-year programme will usually only be agreed for a one-year block (i.e. the second year). Time out of parts of either year will only be considered in exceptional circumstances.

What if your plans change?

If your plans change after time out of the programme has been agreed, the deanery/foundation school will attempt to find a placement for you at short notice but cannot guarantee to do so.

Coming back

If one year out of the programme is agreed, you will, in principle, have the right to return at the end of that year. You will have to take part in the second year allocation process at the same time as other trainees who will be starting their F2 year when you are.

You must inform your FTPD that you are coming back to the programme six months before the start date of your second year placement. You do this by completing your year two preference request. If you don't do this, you won't have a placement arranged within the deanery/foundation school on your return. That means you'll need to go through the competitive application process again for a stand-alone F2 appointment.

Statutory rights

Trainees needing to take time out of programme where statutory employment rights are involved (e.g. maternity and sick leave) have full entitlement to those rights.

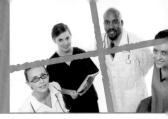

Location

Inter-deanery transfers

If you need to change your deanery from the one that originally accepted you, you should talk to your FTPD. Any transfers will usually take place at the start of either the first or second year.

Arrangements for a transfer must be agreed between postgraduate deans on the basis of well-founded special circumstances.

You will only be able to transfer if:

- you have satisfied both deaneries and foundation schools that you have a good reason for transferring
- there are places available in the receiving deanery/foundation school.

Permanent withdrawal

For those not eligible for an inter-deanery transfer, it is possible (although discouraged) to withdraw from one foundation school in order to complete the second year within another. Before you do this, you should seek counselling and advice from your educational supervisor, foundation training programme director or foundation school director.

If, after discussion, you still wish to withdraw from your foundation school and give up your individual foundation programme, you will need to apply for an advertised stand-alone second year post.

If you are considering this course of action, you should be aware of your professional responsibility to your original employer. Ensure that you give at least the minimum period of notice laid out in your contract, and bear in mind that your employer needs adequate time to make other arrangements to meet patient and service needs.

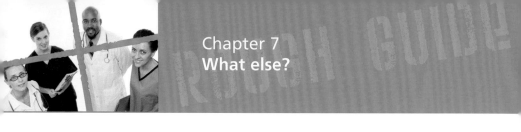

Gaining competences outside the UK

If you take time out of the programme to undertake clinical work/training overseas it is possible that your training could meet the requirements of second year training in the UK. For this, the following conditions may be required:

- it can be demonstrated that the overseas placement will deliver training in the required competences

- the overseas training programme will use the competency-based assessment methods to assess the trainee in accordance with the documentation required by the UK Foundation Programme

- the proposed training programme has been agreed by the postgraduate dean before the trainee takes up the placement.

You should speak to your foundation school director about this in the first instance.

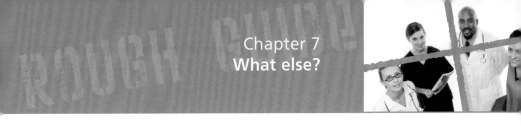
Trainees in difficulty

What if things go wrong?

Sometimes, for some trainees, things will go wrong. For one reason or another, whether because of illness, family pressures, financial stress, or lack of aptitude for medicine as a career, some trainees will fail to progress in the expected way.

The competency assessment process is designed to ensure that any potential problems are identified, and strategies employed to resolve them as soon as possible, at every stage of your training.

The most important thing is recognising when problems are developing and seeking help. It is also important that you engage with the assessment system in a timely manner so that surprises are not stored up until it's too late to do anything about them within the current placement.

Don't worry. You will be supported.

Educational support

There is a range of sources of educational support available to trainees in difficulty. See your educational supervisor who will be able to guide you through the problem or refer you to an appropriate person to speak to. Alternatively, you can speak to the foundation training programme director.

People learn at different rates, and there is nothing wrong with asking for extra help if something is proving difficult. Alternatively, your assessments may reveal areas in which you need support. In this case your educational supervisor will draw your attention to the need for extra educational support, perhaps in the form of intensified experience or supervision.

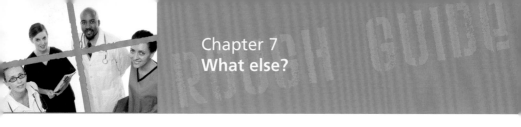

What happens if you fail?

If, for one reason or another, you are not be able to demonstrate the required level of competence:

In the first year (or equivalent for those training less than full-time)
If you fail in the first year, you will not be granted full registration with the GMC and will not be able to progress to F2.

You will be given remedial support for up to one additional year. If, at the end of this time, you still do not meet the required standards, you would be expected to stop practising medicine.

In the second year (or equivalent for those training less than full-time)
In the first instance, remedial training placement will be arranged for a fixed period, usually six months. Exceptionally, one further fixed-term extension may be agreed to a maximum of a further six months.

If you still cannot demonstrate the required level of competence by the end of the second year, you will not receive a Foundation Achievement of Competency Document (FACD).

Other issues requiring support

Psychological support

Medicine is an inherently stressful profession. The first year or two of practice are known to be tough for all but the most resilient of trainees.

It is common, from time to time, to experience feelings of inadequacy or anxiety, and to wonder whether going into medicine was a mistake. Most doctors cope with the stresses of the job by talking over their experiences and feelings with friends, family or peers at work.

Your educational supervisor will also be able to offer support, either directly or by suggesting a colleague to talk to. Many hospitals and deaneries offer a confidential counselling service, contact details of which are likely to be posted in the education centre, or included in the induction pack.

The BMA also provides a 24-hour counselling service which can be contacted on 08459 200169.

Remember, you are not alone.

For professional, ethical and personal matters, support is available.

- **Professional**: Talking to colleagues would be appropriate depending on the situation, as would approaching a senior member of staff.

  For serious professional matters, discussion with a professional advisor such as the services provided by the BMA or a defence organisation would be the safest and most appropriate route.

- **Ethical**: The BMA has an ethics department. If there is a serious ethical issue you should contact the BMA on 020 7383 6286, or the GMC which also provides advice to doctors on professional ethics. Many hospitals now have a clinical ethics committee which could be accessed following advice from the educational supervisor.

- **Personal**: For personal matters, most people turn to their peers, family or friends. If however there is a problem that may impact on your work, it is wise to discuss it with a senior colleague such as your educational supervisor. The BMA provides a confidential counselling service available 24 hours a day. The service is run by professional counsellors and provides help for BMA members and their families on personal, emotional and work-related problems. Just call 08459 200169.

Health support

It is one of your duties as a doctor to take care of your own health but it is all too easy to become physically run down.

It is hard to find time to access and eat a balanced diet, and shift work leads to upset diurnal rhythms and sleep deprivation. Pre-existing conditions may be aggravated by the lifestyle.

Working through illness, self-prescription and the use of alcohol or other substances to relieve stress are risky for you and your patients. Don't do it. Doctors whose health or behaviour might put patients at risk will be referred to the GMC.

That's why you should register with a general practitioner near where you live or work and seek their advice when unwell. Occupational health services are provided within each hospital and are another source of support and advice.

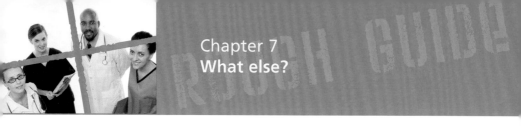

Employment support

Check with your HR department if you have any questions about your contract, hours of employment, salary, appropriateness of duties, and any bullying or harassment issues.

The deanery/foundation school and the employing trust have a responsibility to ensure that the bullying or harassment of trainees by anyone involved in their training or working environment is not tolerated. Both the deanery/foundation school and the trust will have a policy on bullying and harassment that you should be made aware of.

Further contractual and employment information is available to you in the BMA's Junior Doctors' Handbook (www.bma.org.uk) and from askBMA on the number below.

Numbers to call for help

- askBMA: 0870 606 0828, 8am – 6pm, M-F
- BMA 24-hour counselling service: 08459 200169
- GMC: 0845 357 3456
- Medical Defence Union: 0800 716 646 (24/7 emergency helpline)
- Medical Protection Society: 0845 605 4000 (24/7 emergency helpline)

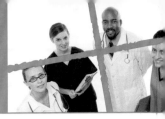

Who's who?

A whole variety of key people and organisations are referred to throughout the Rough Guide. Below is an explanation of what they do.

Clinical supervisor

Your clinical supervisor is the professional responsible for teaching and supervising you.

Your clinical supervisor is responsible for:

- supervising your day to day clinical and professional practice
- supporting your assessment process
- ensuring that you have the appropriate range and mix of clinical exposures
- arranging a work programme to enable you to attend fixed educational sessions.

You will have at least one named clinical supervisor, known to you, in each training placement. You will be told the name and contact details of your clinical supervisor at the start of your placement.

Educational supervisor

Your educational supervisor is the doctor responsible for making sure you receive appropriate training and experience. They will also decide whether individual placements have been completed.

The educational supervisor must be involved in teaching and training, and should help your professional and personal development. Your educational supervisor is responsible for:

- undertaking regular formative appraisal
- providing support so you can develop your learning portfolio
- ensuring you understand and engage in assessment
- being the first point of call for your concerns/issues about training
- ensuring appropriate training opportunities are available for you to learn and gain competences.

You will have a named educational supervisor for each placement. You will be told their name and contact details of their educational supervisor at the start of your placement.

Your clinical supervisor and educational supervisor could be the same person, or two separate people.

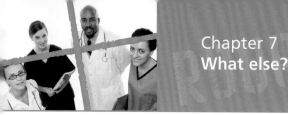

Foundation training programme director (FTPD)

An FTPD is the individual appointed by the deanery and trust to manage and lead a foundation training programme.

Clinical tutor (director of medical education)

The clinical tutor, sometimes also known as director of medical education, is the individual appointed by the postgraduate dean and the trust to manage postgraduate medical education within the trust. It is their responsibility, on behalf of the dean, to ensure that the learning environment within the trust supports the provision of high quality postgraduate medical education and training. They provide professional leadership and vision for the organisation on medical education issues and work closely with the postgraduate dean and foundation school to develop the team of consultants and other health professionals that are responsible for supporting elements of the Foundation Programme as well as the provision of specialty training.

Foundation schools

Foundation schools are not bricks and mortar institutions, but rather a conceptual grouping of institutions, which is administered by an actual (rather than conceptual) staff. The foundation school staff brings together medical schools, the local deanery, trusts (acute, mental health and PCTs) and other organisations (e.g. hospices) to offer you training in a range of different settings and clinical environments.

They offer all the placements you need to gain the competences required to become a fully qualified doctor, as set out in the curriculum.

Foundation schools set up in the UK to accommodate several hundred F1 and F2 doctors each. The schools have a number of foundation training programmes, each under the supervision of a foundation training programme director (FTPD). Each FTPD will have responsibility for 20 – 40 foundation doctors.

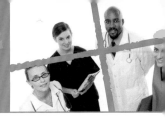

Foundation Doctor Centred Training

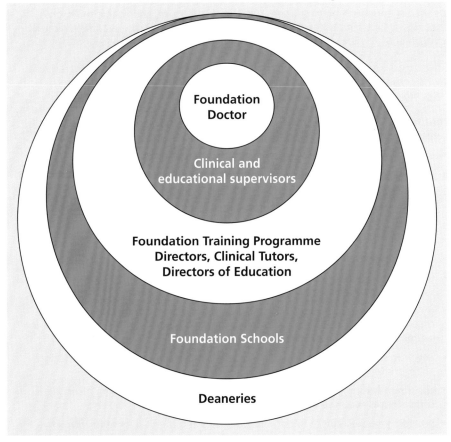

The entire programme is centred around the foundation doctor, who is supported through clinical and educational supervisors. They, in turn, are supported by FTPDs, clinical tutors and directors of education, who are supported by the foundation school structure. All of this is supported by and overseen by the deaneries/foundation schools.

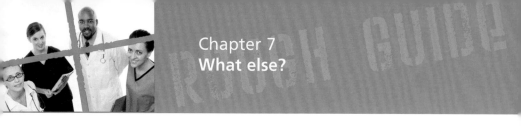

Postgraduate deaneries

Deaneries engage in arrangements with local NHS trusts and others to ensure that trusts, GP training practices and health authorities provide a suitable learning environment to meet the requirements of general medical and specialist training.

There are 14 postgraduate deaneries in England, each headed by a postgraduate dean. They have operational responsibility for ensuring that the Foundation Programme is delivered to national standards set by the GMC and the PMETB. They are responsible for ensuring there is an effective educational infrastructure for foundation training through the foundation schools. In particular, they are responsible for:

- information about and recruitment to the Foundation Programme
- shadowing arrangements in some parts of the country and induction (together with the NHS trust)
- ensuring that local assessment procedures are in accordance with wider national procedures
- ensuring that appraisal is undertaken regularly and appropriately
- training individuals that undertake assessments
- through the foundation training programme director, identifying an educational supervisor for each trainee within a Foundation Programme
- through the foundation training programme director, ensuring that trainees' regular appraisals take place and that Learning and Development Portfolios are supported within the process
- ensuring smooth progression of trainees from year one to year two, offering appropriate career management and development opportunities
- ensuring that individual trainees receive the training necessary to meet the competences required
- providing careers advice (along with the NHS and medical schools/university).

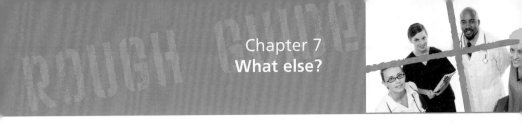

Undergraduate dean/medical school

Medical schools are responsible for confirming that their medical graduates meet the GMC requirements outlined in *Tomorrow's Doctors* for provisional registration.

In accordance with GMC requirements, they are responsible for issuing graduates with written approval to apply for and accept a place in a foundation training programme.

Although medical schools have a statutory responsibility for the PRHO year, in most deaneries this responsibility is given to other organisations, including the postgraduate deanery, the employing NHS trusts or the GMC. Foundation Schools will be organisations which help support joint working with the Postgraduate Deaneries, Medical School, NHS organisations and other healthcare providers.

General Medical Council (GMC)

The GMC has legal powers to protect, promote and maintain the health and safety of the community by ensuring proper standards in the practice of medicine.

To do this, the GMC document *The New Doctor 2007* outlines the required competences to be gained in foundation year one before full registration can be granted.

The GMC also has a responsibility to:

- co-ordinate all stages and promote high standards of medical education
- provisionally register graduates of UK medical schools
- publish guidance on general clinical training and ensure that these guidelines are implemented
- grant full registration to doctors who have gained the required competences
- maintain a list and publish a register of specialist doctors and, in future, a list of general practitioners
- recognise the qualifications awarded by other EEA member states to EEA nationals.

More information can be found at www.gmc-uk.org or by calling 0845 357 8001.

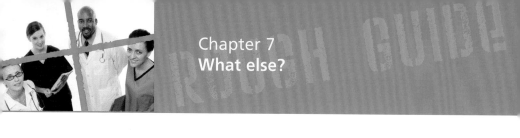

Postgraduate Medical Education and Training Board (PMETB)

The Postgraduate Medical Education and Training Board (PMETB) has a duty to establish, maintain, and develop standards and requirements relating to postgraduate medical education and training in the UK.

The PMETB's remit covers higher and specialist training for doctors. It develops and assesses the standards for training to be delivered by the F2 year and beyond.

PMETB went live on 30 September 2005. It approves the post-F1 training of doctors and certifies that doctors have reached a level of competence required for inclusion in the Specialist/GP Register. More information can be found at www.pmetb.org.uk.

Medical royal colleges and faculties

There are medical royal colleges and faculties for all medical specialties including general practice. The role of individual colleges and faculties is to develop and advise the Postgraduate Medical Education and Training Board (PMETB) regarding the curriculum for each medical specialty.

In advising and supporting the PMETB they:

- publish curricula which identifies the knowledge, skills and attitudes required within each specialty
- recommend to the PMETB the awarding or withholding of educational approval posts, placements and programmes
- determine the standards of professional education and training through examinations/assessments that trainees must pass
- support the delivery of training programmes through regular inspection of approved posts, placement and programmes

The contact information for each medical royal college can be found by going to www.aomrc.org.uk or by calling 020 7692 3197.

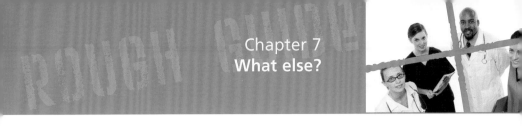
The UK Foundation Programme Office (UKFPO)

The UK Foundation Programme Office will provide a central information point for medical schools, foundation schools, foundation trainees and the faculty involved in foundation training. The aim of the UKFPO is to develop and promote innovative training methods, such as e-learning and the electronic portfolio, as well as to develop and administer the recruitment and programme allocation system throughout England, Northern Ireland, Wales and Scotland.

For more information go to www.foundationprogramme.nhs.uk.

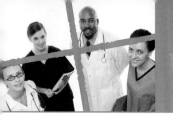
Healthcare organisations/employers

In England, these are NHS trusts which comprise hospitals and groups of general practices that provide healthcare services.

They have employer responsibilities for you during your foundation training.

This means that they will:

- issue you with a contract of employment
- meet the terms and conditions of doctors in training, including hours of work and payment for banding arrangements
- ensure that postgraduate education is delivered and supports learning and meets required educational standards
- ensure a safe working environment
- protect you and all from bullying and harassment
- provide an environment which respects diversity and equality of opportunity
- undertake disciplinary action with respect to contract and performance (although disciplinary procedures for doctors in training are primarily the responsibility of postgraduate deans)
- support the training of trainers.

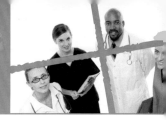

Further information

Foundation Programme Curriculum

The curriculum sets outs the educational content of the two year Foundation Programme. It defines the skills, knowledge and attributes that trainees should demonstrate they have attained. All trainees will be formally assessed during the F1 and F2 years on the competences contained in the curriculum. The curriculum is available electronically on the UKFPO website www.foundationprogramme.nhs.uk.

The curriculum is a working document. Should you have any feedback for the next revision, please email: Chair of the AoMRC Foundation Committee at foundationcommittee@aomrc.org.uk

Or write to:
Chair of the Foundation Committee
Academy of Medical Royal Colleges
1 Wimpole Street
London
W1G 0AW

Operational Framework for Foundation Training

This document supports the implementation of foundation training programmes and is designed for use by postgraduate deaneries, clinical tutors, local trusts and foundation school staff. The principles outlined in the framework apply to all countries in the UK, but may be adapted for local circumstances. The Operational Framework can be accessed through the UKFPO website at www.foundationprogramme.nhs.uk.

The Operational Framework is a working document and we welcome your feedback. Should you have any feedback for the next revision, please write to our Operational Framework Co-ordinator at administrator@foundationprogramme.nhs.uk.